This journal

belongs

to:

_____

A DAILY PRESCRIPTION FOR NATURAL HEALTH:
A Journal for Kelee® Meditation Students
A 10-Week Course

This book is an original publication of Quiescence Publishing

PRINTING HISTORY
first edition / October 2016

www.thekelee.org
ISBN: 978-0-9973002-5-3

PRINTED IN THE UNITED STATES OF AMERICA

How to Use This Journal

In this journal you can write your experiences and record your progress. You think you will remember everything, but I can assure you, you will forget many subtle gems of wisdom about how you have grown.

You can draw or write inside the lines, or outside them. You can use pen, pencil, colored pencils, crayons or whatever medium will record what you have experienced, after your Kelee meditation practice. If something is deeply personal to you, only record it, if you would allow another to see it.

If you want to record personal thoughts, write them in such a way, that they would only mean something to you. This journal will be a record of the contents of your mind, and your evolution over time.

—Author, Ron W. Rathbun

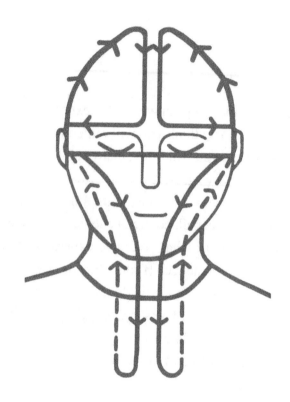

Date: _____ AM / PM

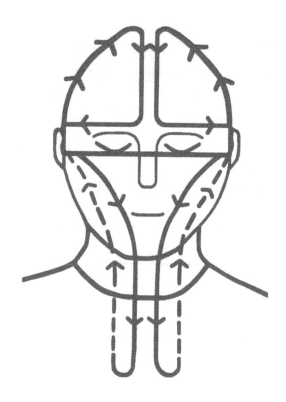

Date: _____ AM / PM

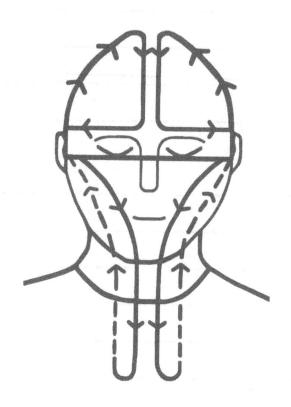

Date: _____ AM / PM

_____

_____

_____

_____

_____

_____

_____

_____

_____

_____

_____

_____

_____

_____

_____

_____

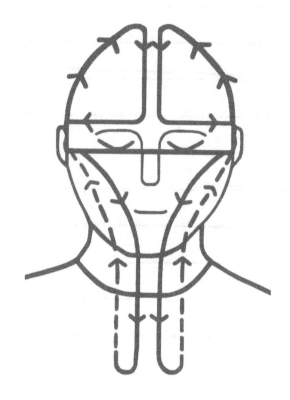

Date: _____ AM / PM

_____

_____

_____

_____

_____

_____

_____

_____

_____

_____

_____

_____

_____

_____

_____

_____

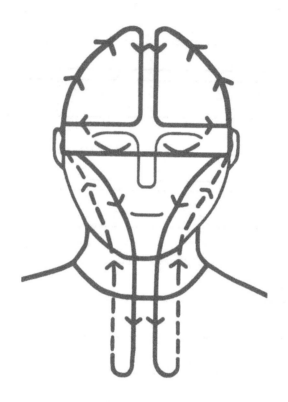

Date: _____ AM / PM

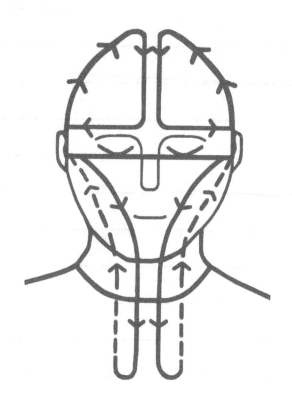

Date: _____ AM / PM

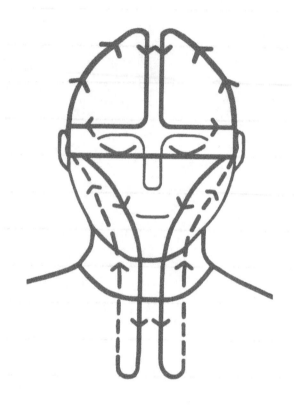

Date: _____ AM / PM

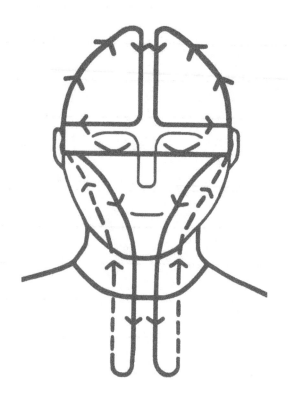

Date: _____ AM / PM

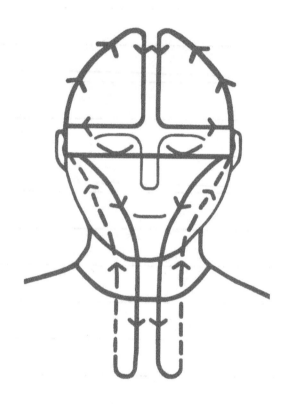

Date: _____ AM / PM

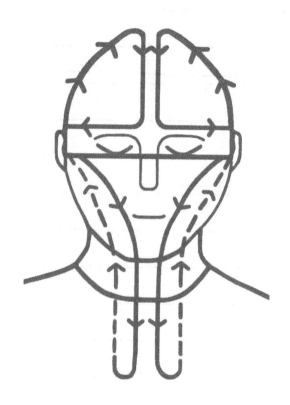

Date: _____ AM / PM

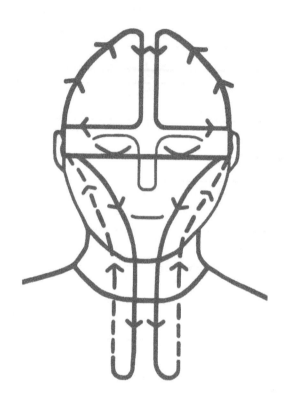

Date: _____ AM / PM

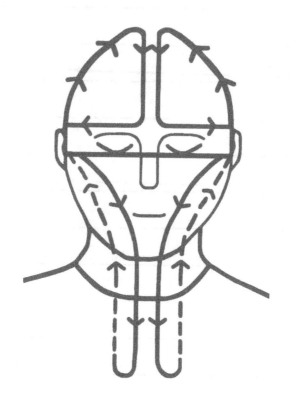

Date: _____ AM / PM

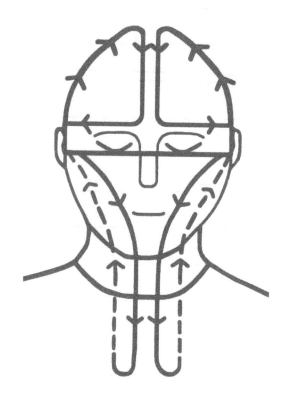

Date: _____ AM / PM

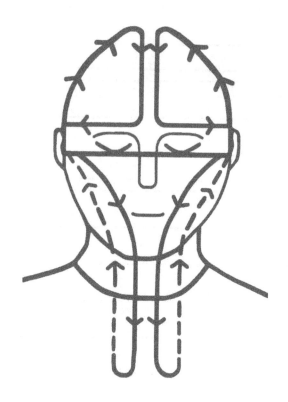

Date: _____ AM / PM

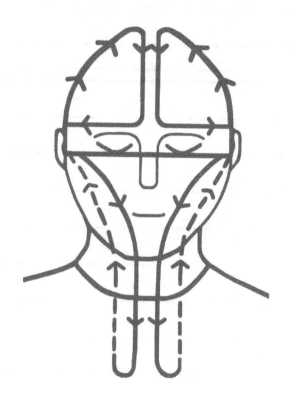

Date: _____ AM / PM

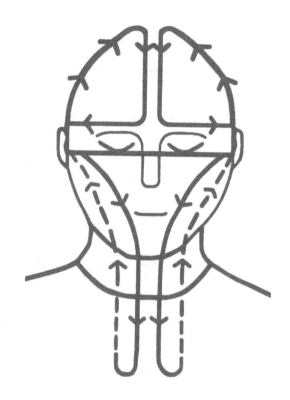

Date: _____ AM / PM

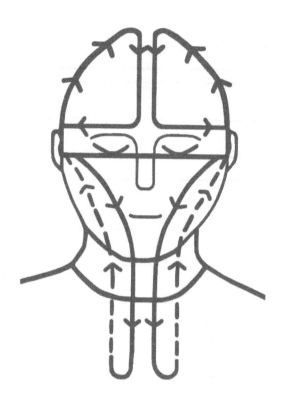

Date: _____ AM / PM

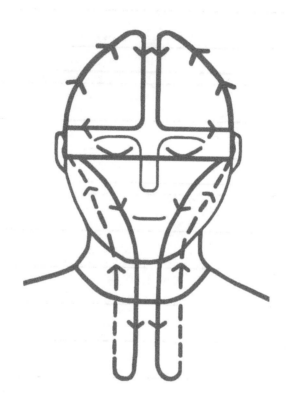

Date: _____ AM / PM

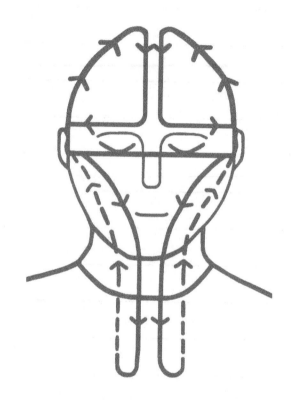

Date: _____ AM / PM

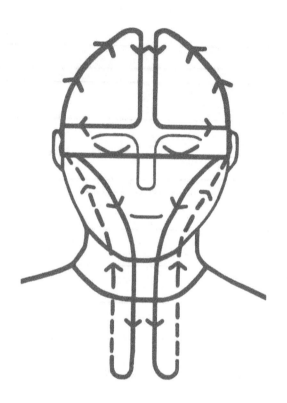

Date: _____ AM / PM

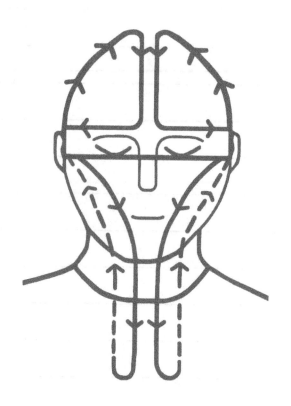

Date: _____ AM / PM

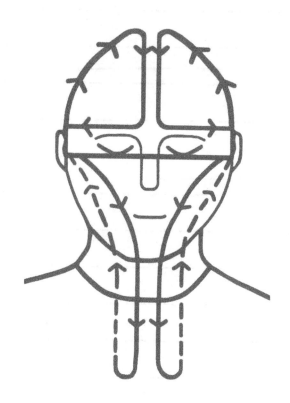

Date: _____ AM / PM

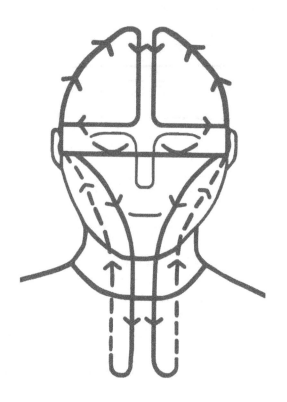

Date: _____ AM / PM

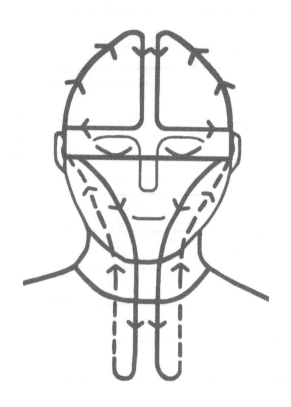

Date: _____ AM / PM

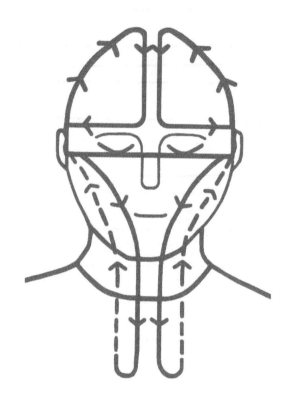

Date: _____ AM / PM

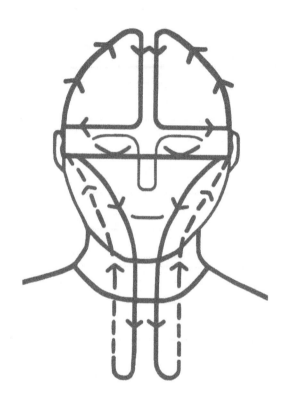

Date: _____ AM / PM

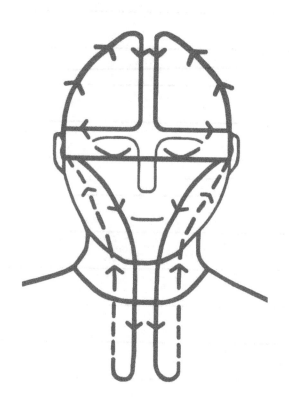

Date: _____ AM / PM

_____

_____

_____

_____

_____

_____

_____

_____

_____

_____

_____

_____

_____

_____

_____

_____

_____

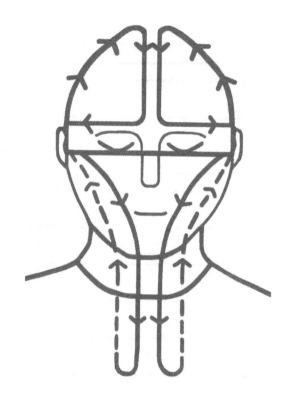

Date: _____ AM / PM

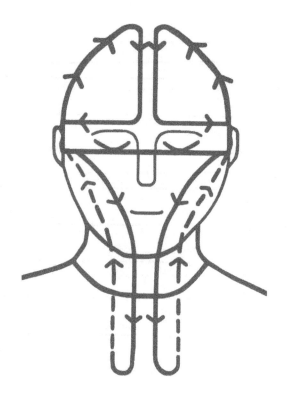

Date: _____ AM / PM

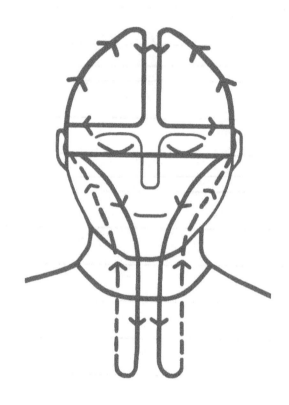

Date: _____ AM / PM

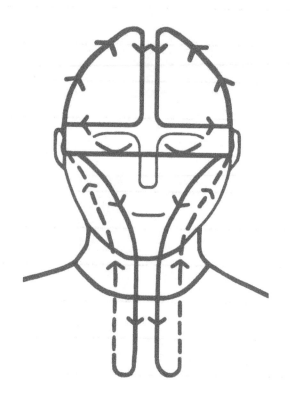

Date: _____ AM / PM

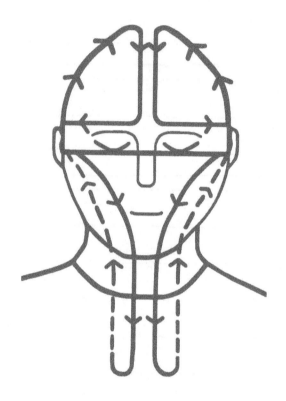

Date: _____ AM / PM

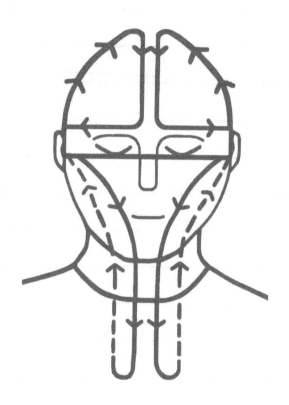

Date: _____ AM / PM

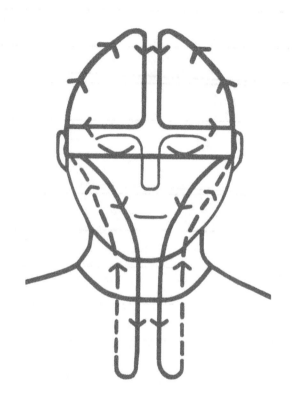

Date: _____ AM / PM

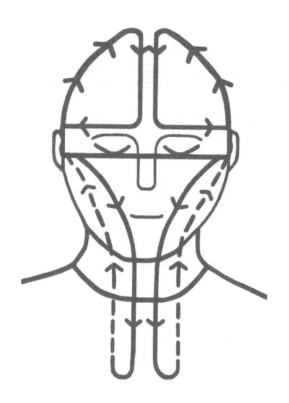

Date: _____ AM / PM

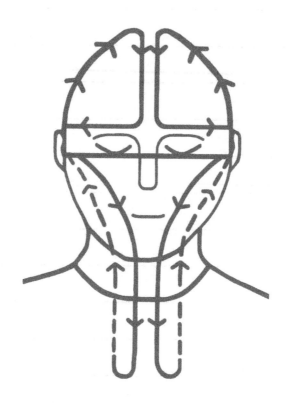

Date: _____ AM / PM

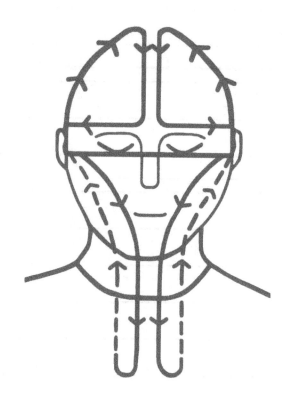

Date: _____ AM / PM

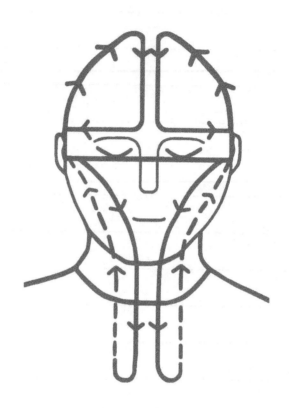

Date: _____ AM / PM

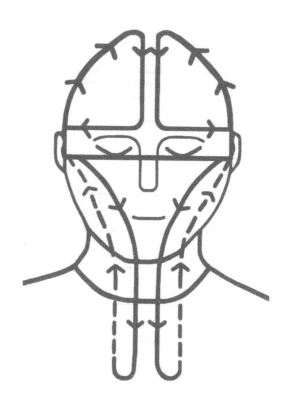

Date: _____ AM / PM

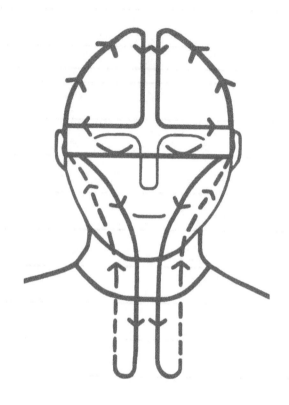

Date: _____ AM / PM

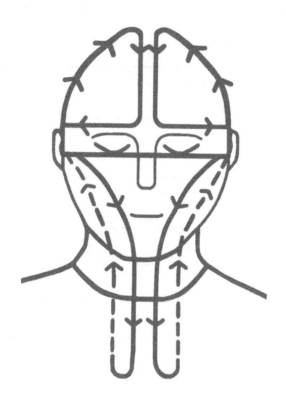

Date: _____ AM / PM

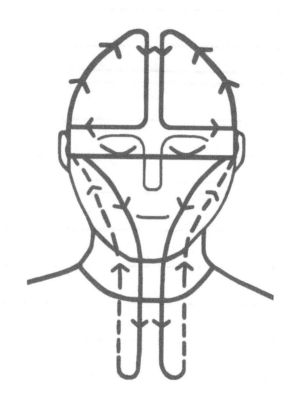

Date: _____ AM / PM

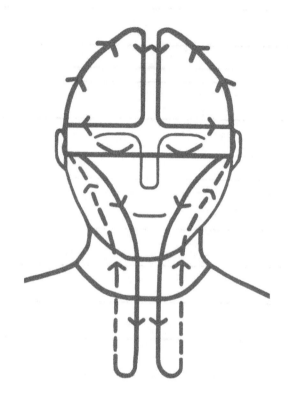

Date: _____ AM / PM

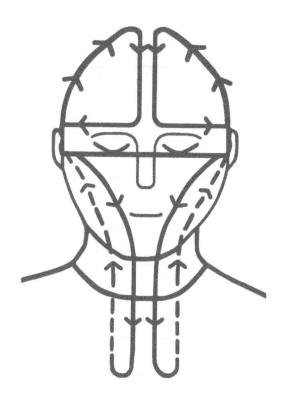

Date: _____ AM / PM

_____

_____

_____

_____

_____

_____

_____

_____

_____

_____

_____

_____

_____

_____

_____

_____

_____

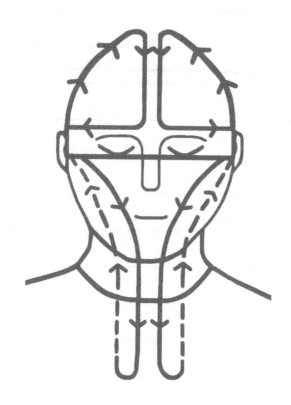

Date: _____ AM / PM

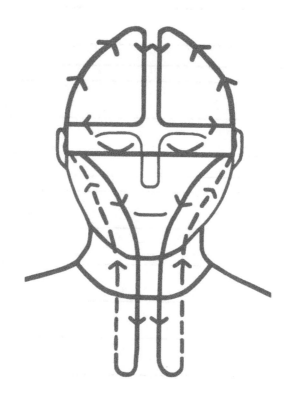

Date: _____ AM / PM

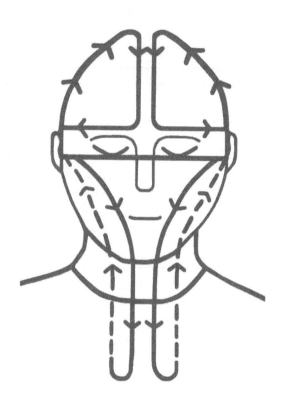

Date: _____ AM / PM

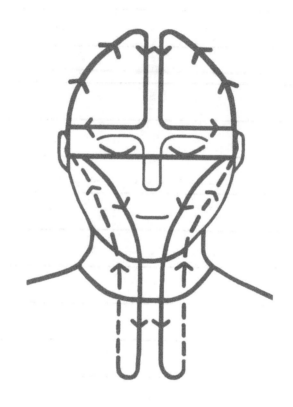

Date: _____ AM / PM

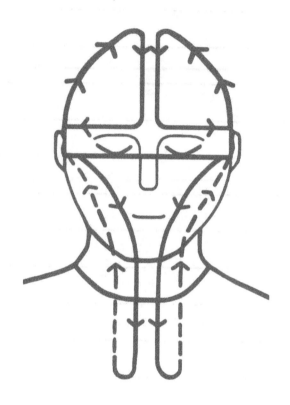

Date: _____ AM / PM

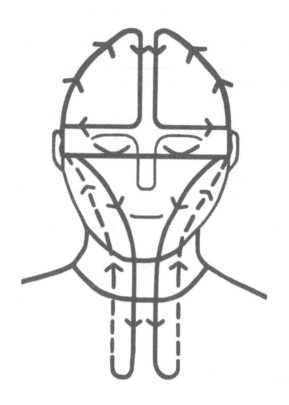

Date: _____ AM / PM

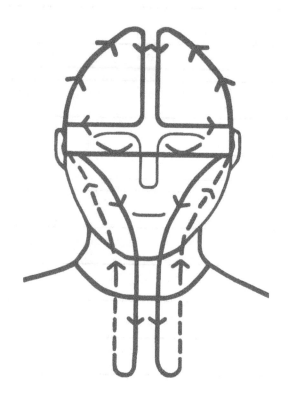

Date: _____ AM / PM

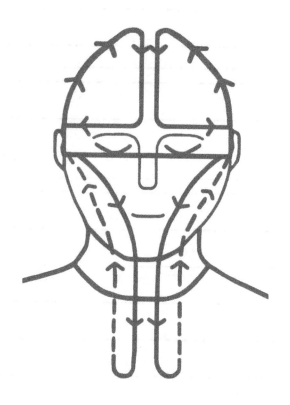

Date: _____ AM / PM

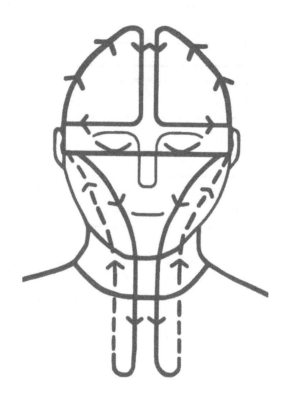

Date: _____ AM / PM

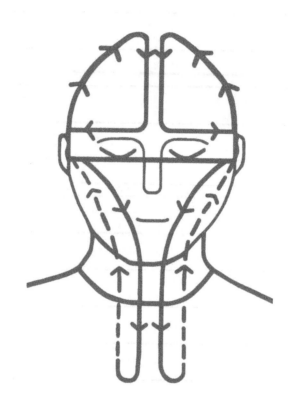

Date: _____ AM / PM

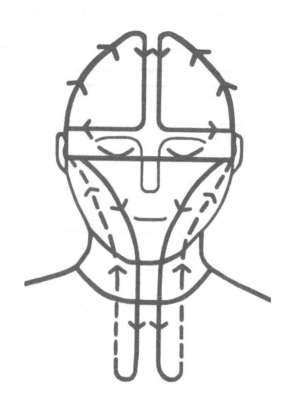

Date: _____ AM / PM

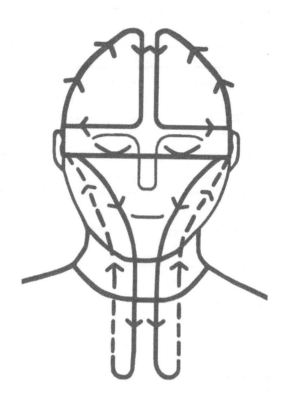

Date: _____ AM / PM

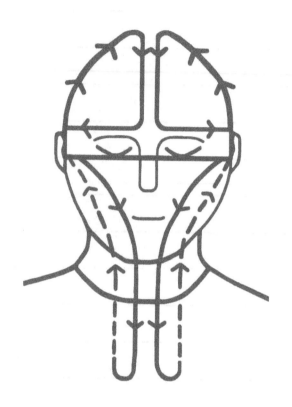

Date: _____ AM / PM

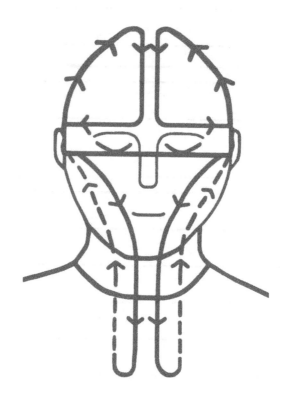

Date: _____ AM / PM

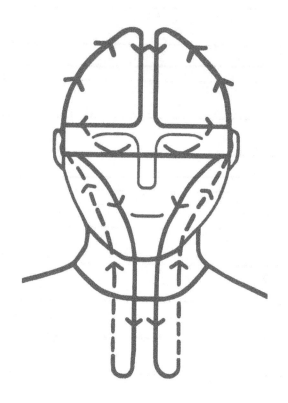

Date: _____ AM / PM

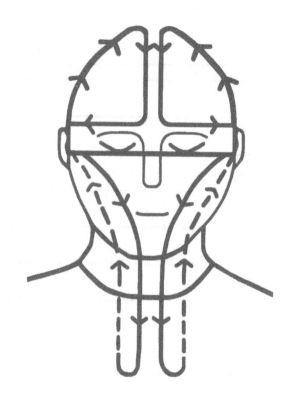

Date: _____ AM / PM

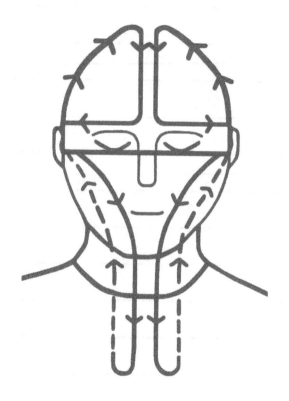

Date: _____ AM / PM

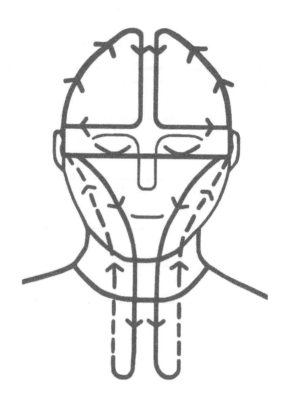

Date: _____ AM / PM

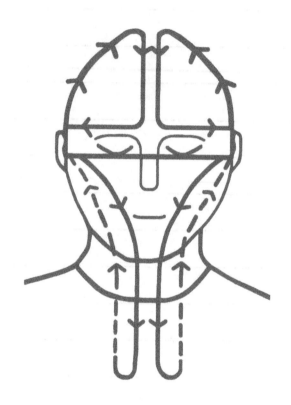

Date: _____ AM / PM

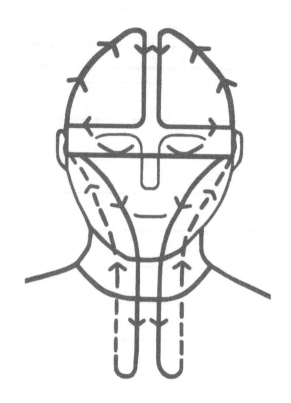

Date: _____ AM / PM

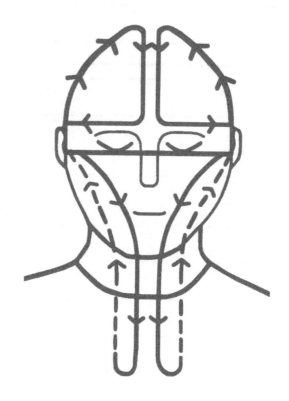

Date: _____ AM / PM

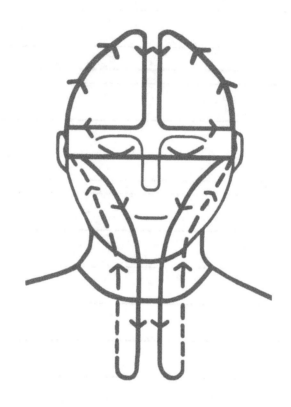

Date: _____ AM / PM

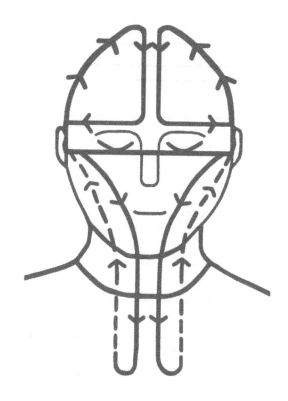

Date: _____ AM / PM

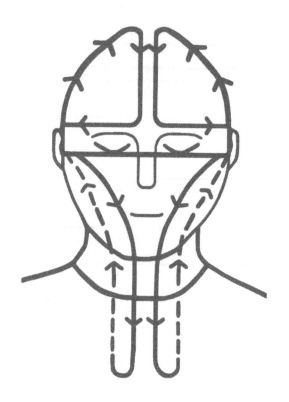

Date: _____ AM / PM

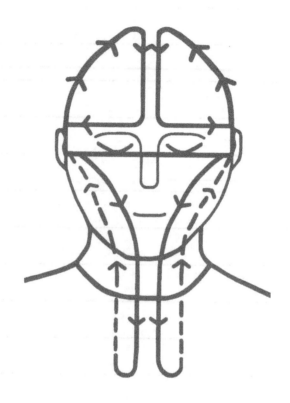

Date: _____ AM / PM

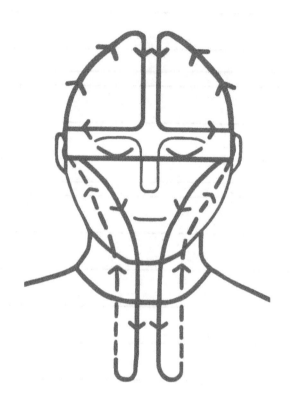

Date: _____ AM / PM

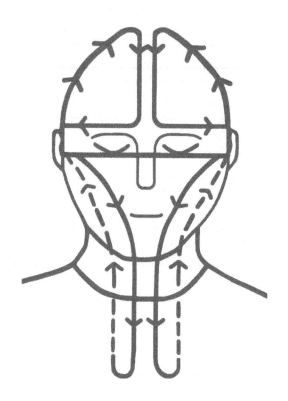

Date: _____ AM / PM

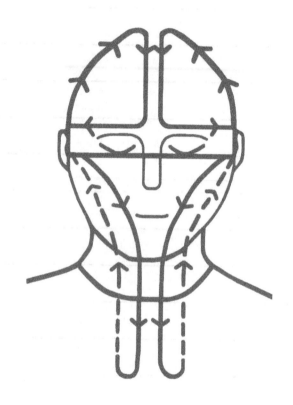

Date: _____ AM / PM

_____

_____

_____

_____

_____

_____

_____

_____

_____

_____

_____

_____

_____

_____

_____

_____

_____

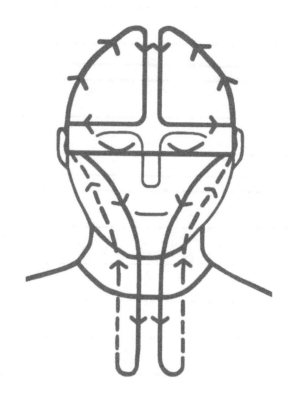

Date: _____ AM / PM

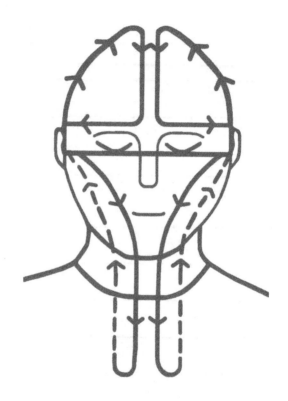

Date: _____ AM / PM

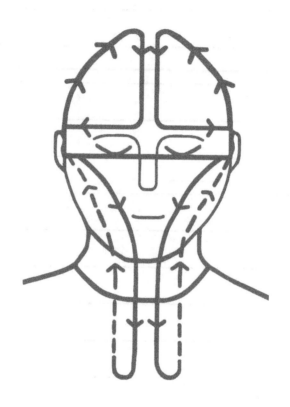

Date: _____ AM / PM

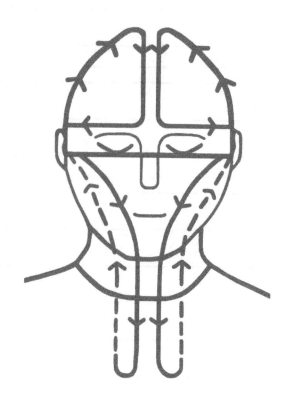

Date: _____ AM / PM

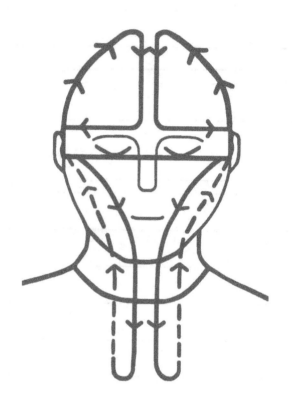

Date: _____ AM / PM

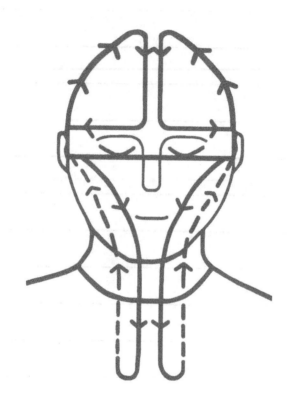

Date: _____ AM / PM

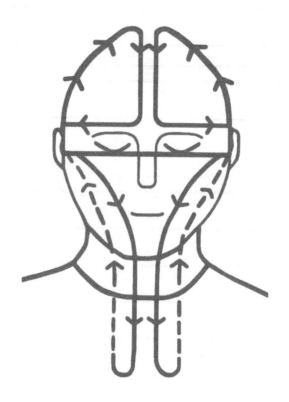

Date: _____ AM / PM

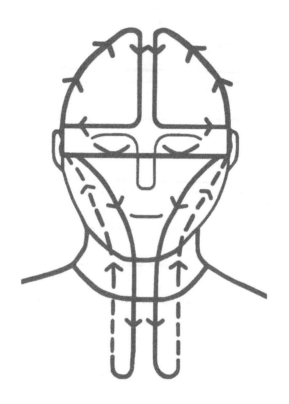

Date: _____ AM / PM

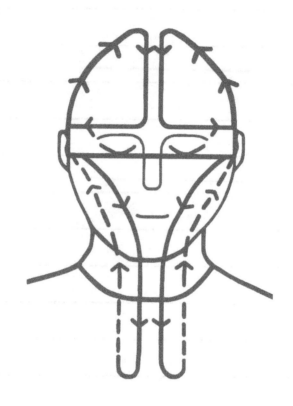

Date: _____ AM / PM

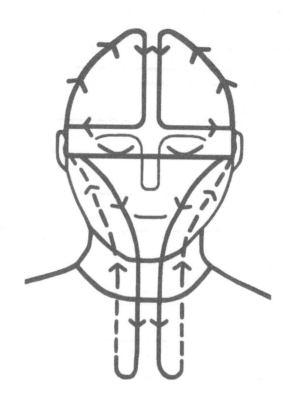

Date: _____ AM / PM

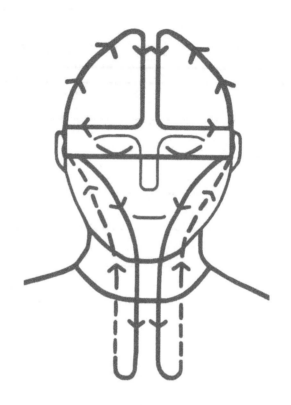

Date: _____ AM / PM

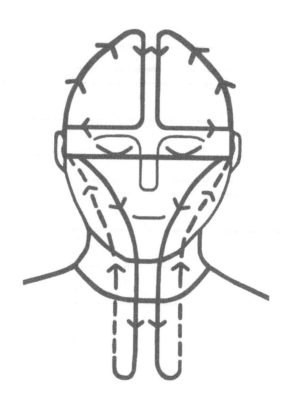

Date: _____ AM / PM

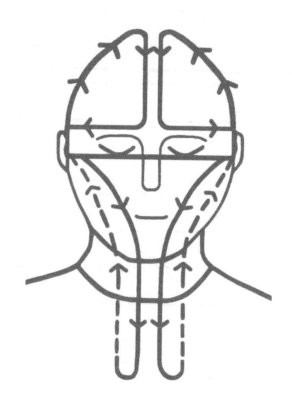

Date: _____ AM / PM

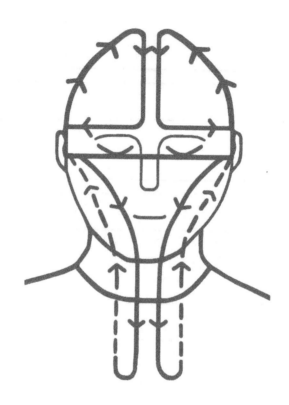

Date: _____ AM / PM

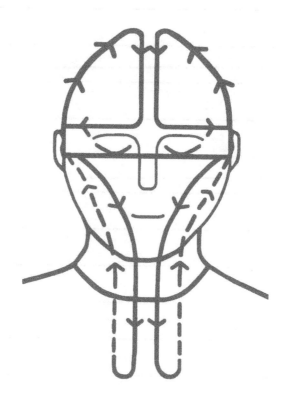

Date: _____ AM / PM

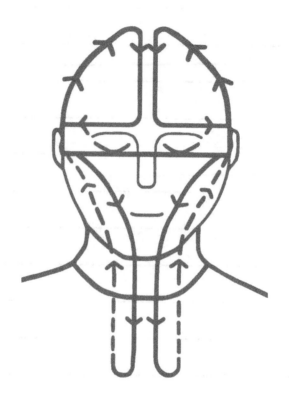

Date: _____ AM / PM

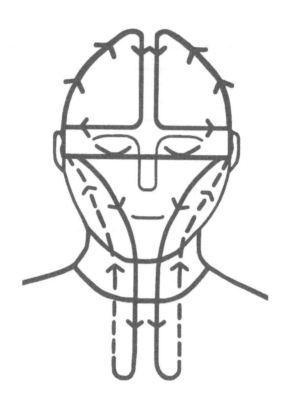

Date: _____ AM / PM

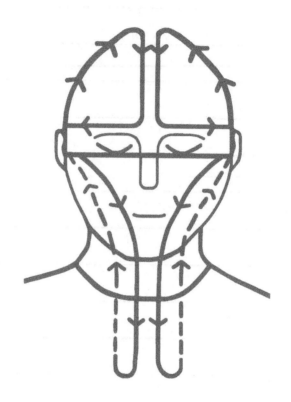

Date: _____ AM / PM

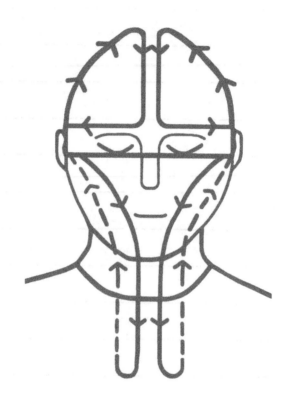

Date: _____ AM / PM

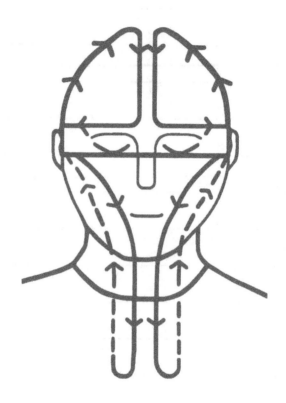

Date: _____ AM / PM

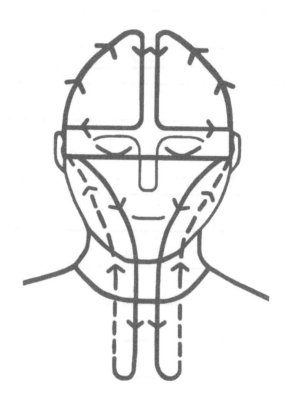

Date: _____ AM / PM

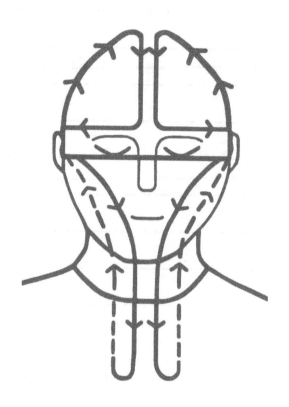

Date: _____ AM / PM

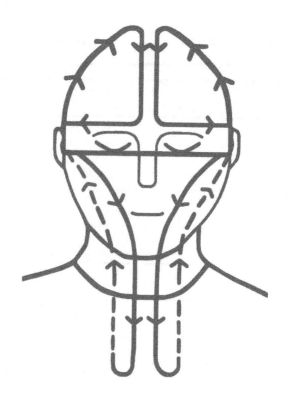

Date: _____ AM / PM

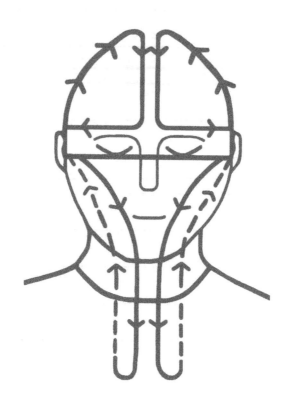

Date: _____ AM / PM

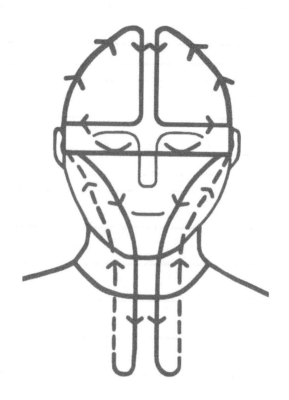

Date: _____ AM / PM

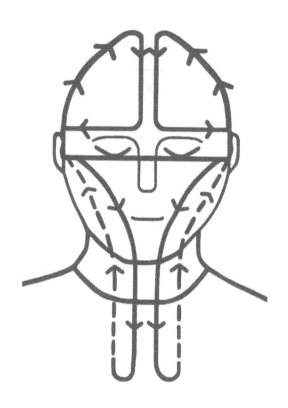

Date: _____ AM / PM

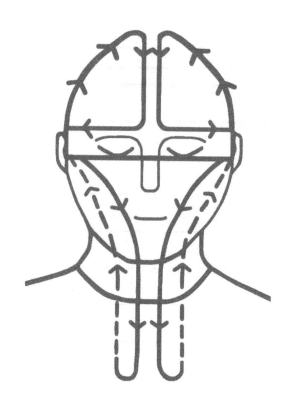

Date: _____ AM / PM

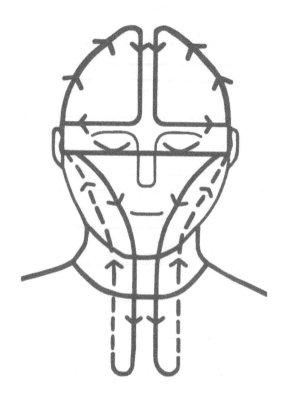

Date: _____ AM / PM

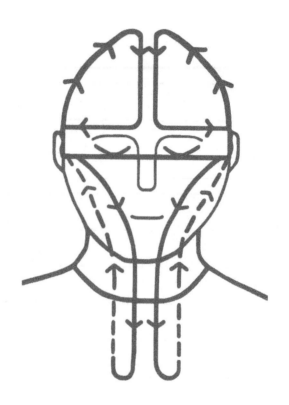

Date: _____ AM / PM

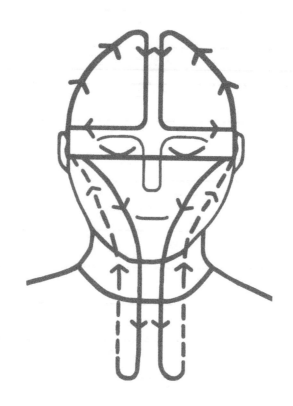

Date: _____ AM / PM

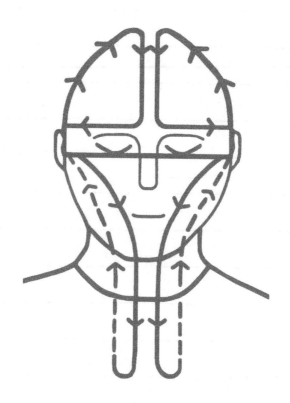

Date: _____ AM / PM

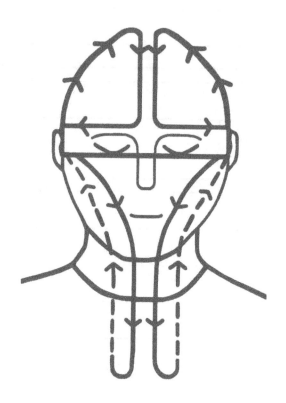

Date: _____ AM / PM

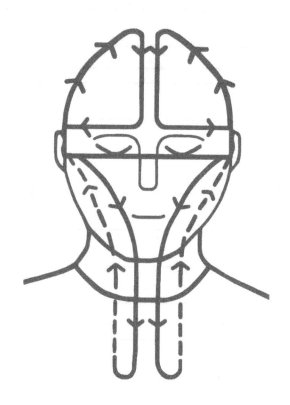

Date: _____ AM / PM

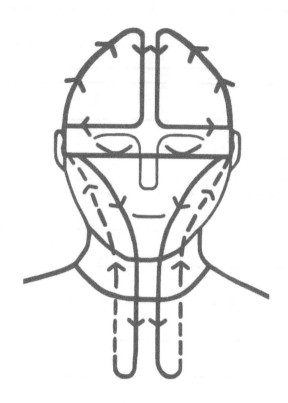

Date: _____ AM / PM

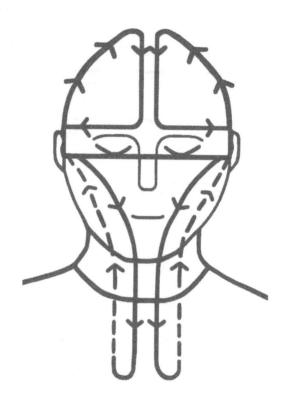

Date: _____ AM / PM

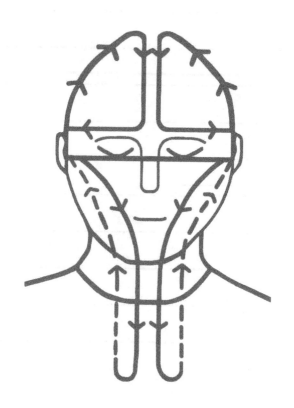

Date: _____ AM / PM

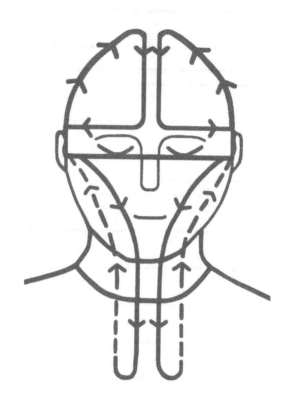

Date: _____ AM / PM

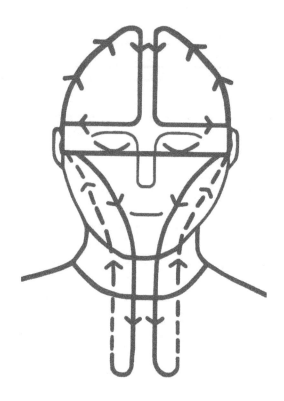

Date: _____ AM / PM

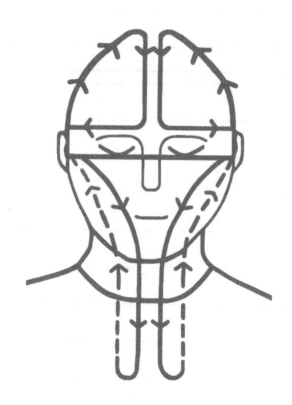

Date: _____ AM / PM

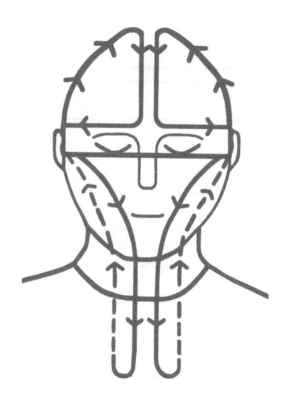

Date: _____ AM / PM

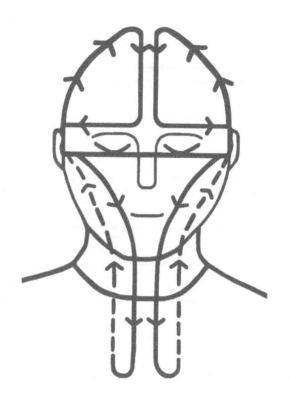

Date: _____ AM / PM

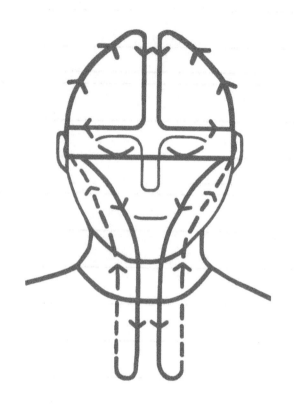

Date: _____ AM / PM

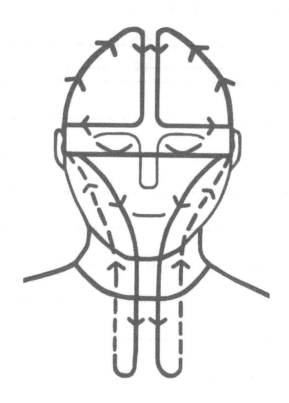

Date: _____ AM / PM

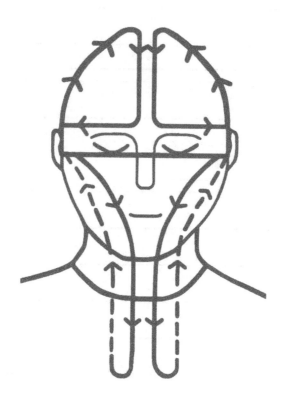

Date: _____ AM / PM

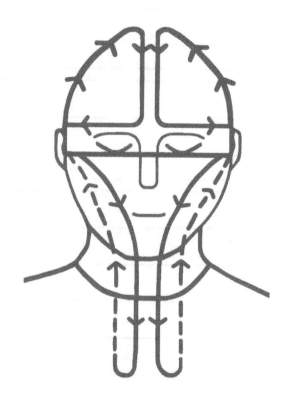

Date: _____ AM / PM

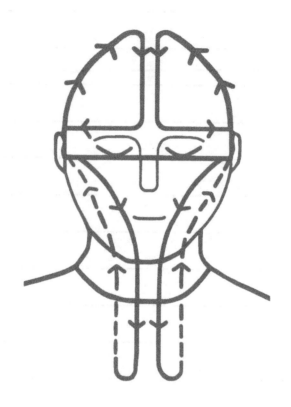

Date: _____ AM / PM

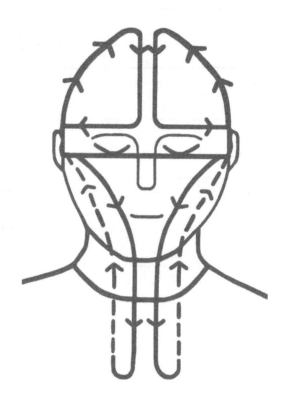

Date: _____ AM / PM

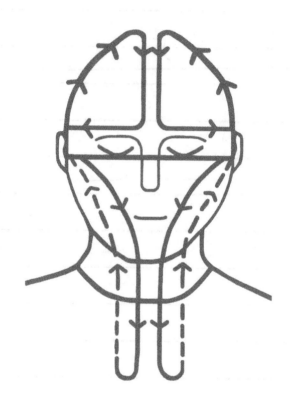

Date: _____ AM / PM

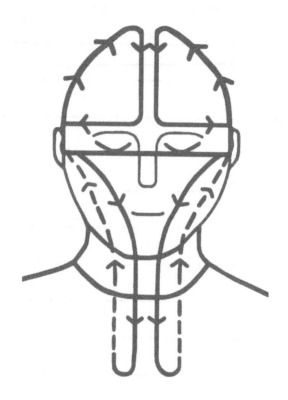

Date: _____ AM / PM

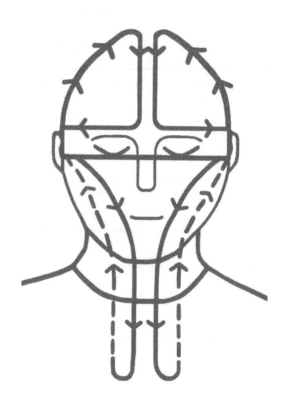

Date: _____ AM / PM

_____

_____

_____

_____

_____

_____

_____

_____

_____

_____

_____

_____

_____

_____

_____

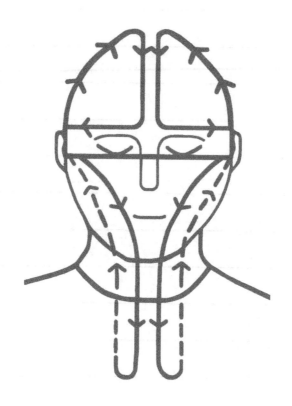

Date: _____ AM / PM

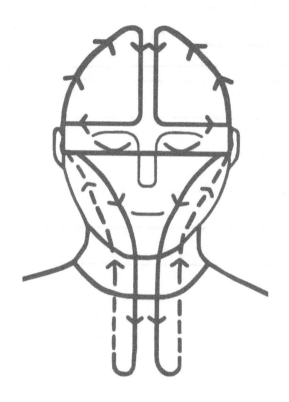

Date: _____ AM / PM

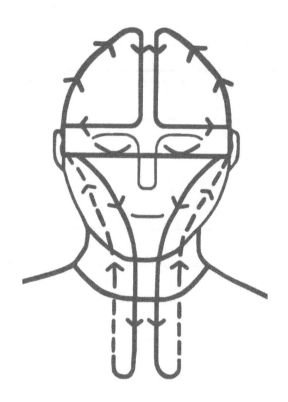

Date: _____ AM / PM

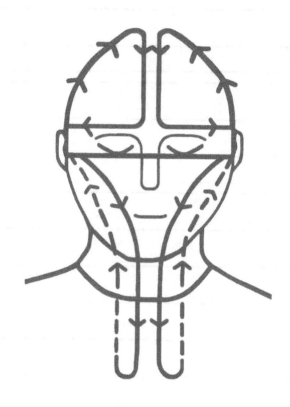

Date: _____ AM / PM

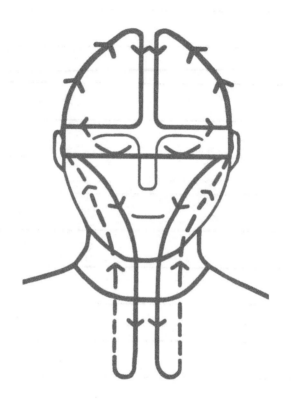

Date: _____ AM / PM

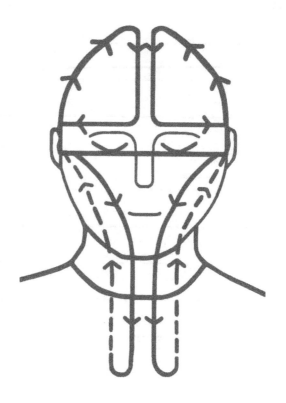

Date: _____ AM / PM

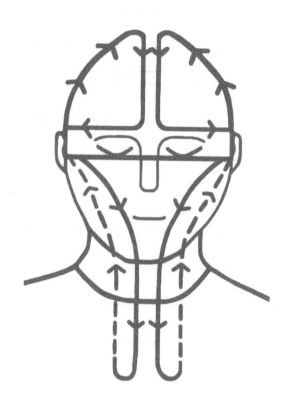

Date: _____ AM / PM

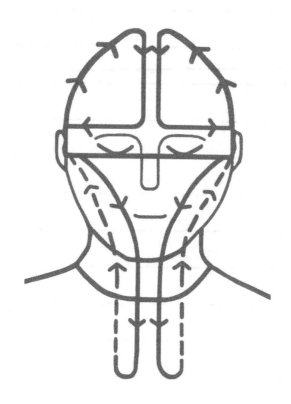

Date: _____ AM / PM

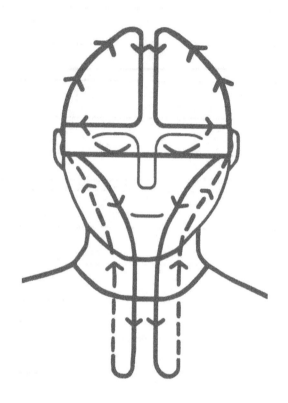

Date: _____ AM / PM

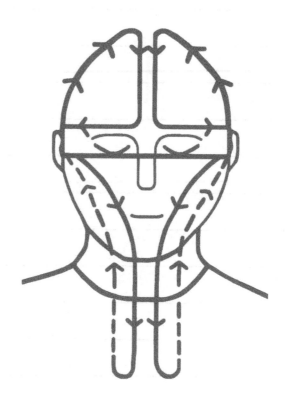

Date: _____ AM / PM

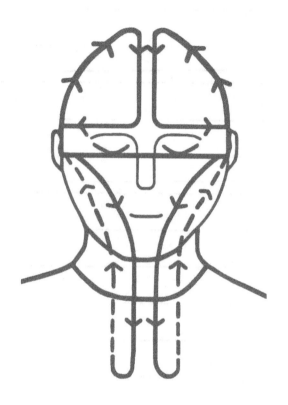

Date: _____ AM / PM

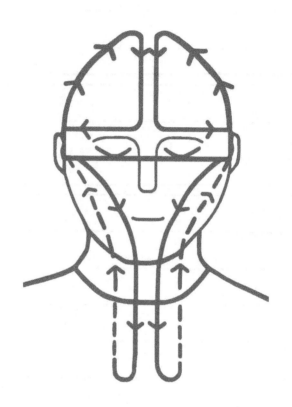

Date: _____ AM / PM

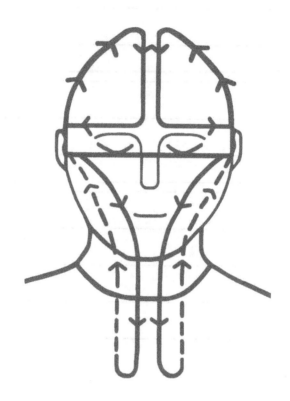

Date: _____ AM / PM

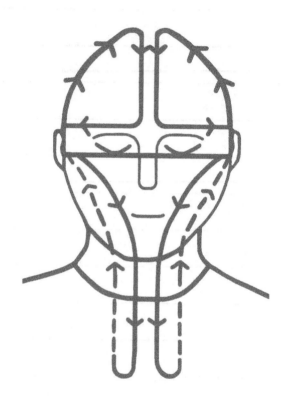

Date: _____ AM / PM

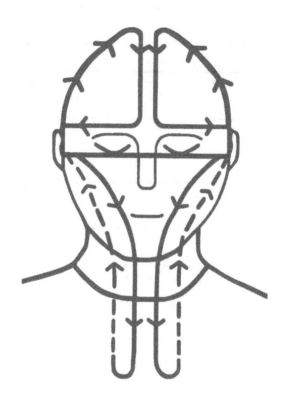

Date: _____ AM / PM

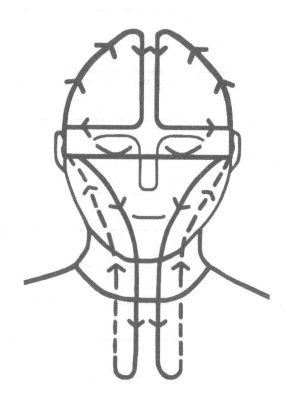

Date: _____ AM / PM

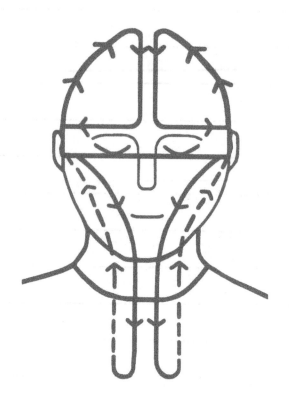

Date: _____ AM / PM

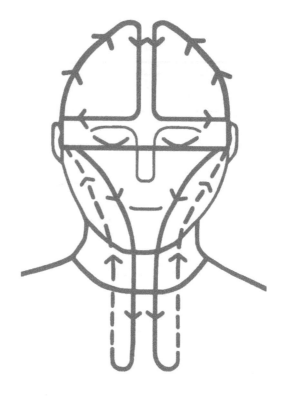

This is the last meditation of this journal.
Now refer back to your first meditation.
How have you changed ...
Keep going!

Date: _____ AM / PM

The Lesser Kelee ⸺⸺⸺⸺⸺⟶

The Surface of the Mind ⸺⸺⸺⟶

The Greater Kelee ⸺⸺⸺⸺⟶

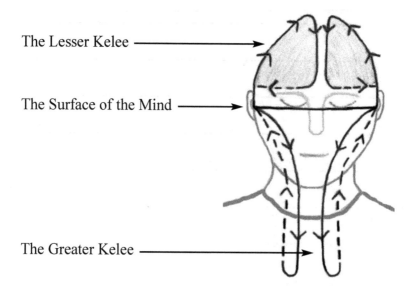

Kelee Meditation

Step One

Approximately two minutes.

Sit down, get comfortable, and begin relaxing your brain activity. Bring your conscious awareness to the top of your head and feel it as a horizontal plane of awareness relaxing down through both hemispheres of your brain to the surface of your mind.

Be consciously relaxed, but not thinking.

Step Two

Approximately three minutes.

Relax and allow your awareness to drop below the surface of your mind into your greater Kelee to a still point within. The goal is to let go of sense consciousness and experience total stillness before returning to full consciousness.

Note: Before you drop from the surface your mind, set your biological clock to bring you back to complete awareness in about three minutes.

Step Three

Approximately five minutes.

Upon returning to the surface of your mind, reflect on what you noticed about your practice. Do not bolt into your day. Pace yourself.

Do your practice for ten minutes in the morning and evening to the best of your ability and get into the experience of your life. Allow the true nature of your being to unfold.

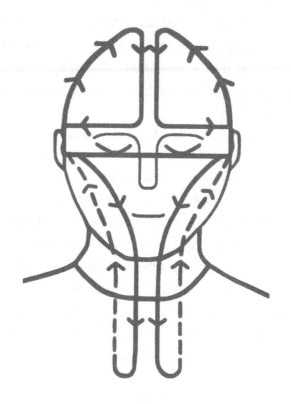

Changes in Your life

To develop clear perception and self-assuredness, here are some thoughts to contemplate.

1. Have people noticed changes in you, and are they treating you differently.

2. Are you feeling less distracted in your mind, by things in your life that do not matter to you personally.

3. Have you noticed a change in how something that has bothered you, or affected you, has lessened.

4. Do you know when you're triggered and looping through compartments, or are you processing out and letting go of compartments.

5. Are you aware of being present with your thoughts, while in your daily activities.

6. Have your views of the world around you changed, and if so, how.

7. How do you feel about yourself, has that changed, and if so how.

8. Have you felt feelings of beauty, freedom, or euphoria for no apparent outside reason.

9. Do you feel more space in your mind, and what does that space feel like.

CPSIA information can be obtained
at www.ICGtesting.com
Printed in the USA
FSHW01n2058250618
49813FS